THE ESSENTIAL GUIDE TO

Natural Pet Care

CANCER

THE ESSENTIAL GUIDE TO

Natural Pet Care

CANCER

CAL OREY

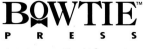

BOWTIE™

P R E S S

Irvine, California

Thanks to the San Carlos Library, San Carlos, California.　　—C.O.

Ruth Berman, editor-in-chief
Nick Clemente, special consultant
Book design and layout by Michele Lanci-Altomare and Victor W. Perry
Mike Uyesugi, cover design

Library of Congress Cataloging-in-Publication Data

Orey, Cal, 1952-
    Cancer / by Cal Orey.
        p.   cm. -- (The essential guide to natural pet care)
    Includes bibliographical references.
    ISBN 1-889540-35-8 (pbk. : alk. paper)
    1. Dogs--Diseases. 2. Cats--Diseases. 3. Cancer in animals.
    4. Holistic veterinary medicine.   I. Title.   II. Series.
SF992.C35074 1998
636.7'0896994--dc21   98-43387
                                                                    CIP

BowTie™ Press
3 Burroughs
Irvine, California 92618

Manufactured in the United States of America
10 9 8 7 6 5 4 3 2 1

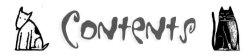

Contents

Foreword   vii

Introduction What Is Cancer?   xi
The Immunity Factor
History of Cancer in Pets
Healing Your Pet with Holistic Medicine

1 Cancer Awareness   1
How to Tell if Your Pet Has Cancer
Symptoms to Look For
Choosing the Right Natural Therapy

2 Natural Therapies   9
Therapy #1: The Health Protection Diet
Therapy #2: Dietary Supplements
Therapy #3: Anticancer Herbs and Homeopathy
Therapy #4: Acupuncture

3 What You Can Do at Home   29
Ten Nondiet Ways to Prevent Cancer

Conclusion What's to Come in the Future   37
The In-Home Computer Revolution
Alternative Therapies on the Rise
A New Wave of Self-Reliance
Life Goes On

Selected Bibliography   43

Complementary medicine (also known as holistic or alternative medicine) has become increasingly popular as an addition to or sometimes even a replacement for conventional medicine. Conventional medicine concentrates on getting immediate results using substances to control a disease process or replace something that is missing. It is invaluable in situations where fast action is imperative, such as surgically removing a cancerous tumor

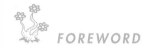

to save a life. Conventional medicine also has diagnostic tools that help us better understand what is going on in the body.

When there is a long-standing problem, when the side effects of conventional medicine are almost as bad as the disease, or when the body isn't functioning quite like it should, holistic medicine often offers a better solution. The approach in holistic medicine is to help the body heal itself with a minimum of side effects. When used to complement conventional medicine, holistic medicine can speed up healing time, decrease side effects, or increase survival time in chronic diseases.

There are probably more misunderstandings about cancer and the roles of conventional and holistic veterinary medicine in preventing and treating cancer than about any other aspect of medicine. In my practice, some pet owners blame themselves for causing cancer in their pets, even if the cancer is caused by factors outside of the owner's control. Other people have such a false sense of security from doing all the "right things" holistically (such as feeding a healthy diet) that they avoid doing things such as spaying or neutering that do far more than a healthy diet does to prevent cancer. A third group is paralyzed by the thought of cancer, and owners in this group can't make up their minds what to do, so they do nothing.

Domesticated dogs and cats are far removed from their wild ancestors. The process of creating any breed makes an animal more inbred than its wild ancestors. Inbreeding increases the occurrence of cancer.

Lifestyle plays as big a part in causing some animal cancers as it does with people. Too much sun can cause skin cancer, and the amount of fat in the diet of dogs has recently been associated with the likelihood of getting mammary tumors. In the wild, animals susceptible to these factors die out and do not produce offspring. In our world of domesticated pets, if the animals are lovable (even if diseased) we keep them, care for them, and breed them for more of the same.

Holistic treatments can help prevent cancer and treat it. Some people don't realize that there are anticancer treatments, rather than "cancer-killer" prevention or treatment methods. These anticancer treatments do not prevent or cure 100 percent of all cases; they just decrease the chances of getting cancer. If you are doing the best you can possibly do, cancer can still appear.

Whether you are preventing or treating cancer, conventional treatments should not be rejected completely. Conventional medicine, especially surgery, often offers enough relief to the body to heal holistically. (This has been experimentally verified in both human and veterinary

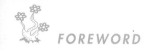
medicine.) While we want to avoid toxic chemicals, and some conventional veterinary treatments may include chemicals with toxic side effects, some conventional methods can greatly decrease the chances of getting cancer. For example, spaying and neutering, even though anesthetics are used, are associated with up to 100 percent less incidence of some types of cancer.

Pet owners can work toward preventing and treating cancer by reading up on the best methods and treatments available. Books such as this one with in-depth research that is cross-checked with a holistic practitioner offer good guidelines for doing just that.

—*Nancy Scanlan, D.V.M.*

What Is Cancer?

On top of Mt. Tamalpais, in southern Marin County, California, lives a pack of Siberian huskies and their devoted owner, Del Goetz. Over the years, these easy-to-love dogs endured an unforgettable tragedy. The feisty gang of nine was hit by deadly hemangiosarcoma—a fast spreading malignant cancer that causes tumors and internal bleeding. Sadly, three Siberians, Wolf, Big Goldie, and Little Goldie, died. Although Del's dog pack is at a higher risk, no dog is immune to cancer.

The statistics on cancer are sobering. More than 50 percent of dogs and cats over ten years of age receive this earth-shattering diagnosis. But as frightening as this may seem, pet owners are not powerless. They don't have to wait for fate to randomly deal their pets a bad hand. There are steps pet owners can take to prevent cancer and steps they can take to cure it naturally. One of the most important steps is to adopt a cancer-fighting plan.

The quality of your pet's diet and lifestyle is an important element in preventing and treating cancer. Cancer treatments can help boost quality and length of life and even cure the disease. To determine the best anti-cancer strategy, we consulted with holistic veterinarians who fight cancer with natural programs. Here, they share the basis for their disease-fighting regimens.

Experts classify cancer as an uncontrolled growth of cells on or within the body. It may be localized (harmless and benign), or it may invade adjacent tissue and spread throughout the body (malignant). In other words, cancer is caused by a mass of toxins that attack an immune system. When enough toxins build up, the system can no longer recognize abnormal cells when they develop. The body then begins to overload on toxins.

"Cancer is the ultimate toxic condition; if proper detoxification is not achieved, that patient will die," says Bob Goldstein, V.M.D., of Westport, Connecticut, veteran holistic practitioner and medical editor of the *Love of Animals* newsletter, published by Earth Animal.

THE IMMUNITY FACTOR

The right foods and lifestyle can strengthen the immune system and ward off illness and disease in humans. Therefore, it's no surprise that a strong immune system helps prevent disease, particularly cancer, in cats and dogs. The immune system's job is to attack and destroy damaged or mutated cells.

"The only time your pet can get cancer is when its body has gone haywire and its immune system is shot," says Pedro Rivera, D.V.M., a holistic vet who specializes in cancer therapy in Sturtevant, Wisconsin.

"Cancer doesn't just happen," says San Francisco–based holistic veterinarian Cheryl Schwartz in her book *Four Paws, Five Directions: A Guide to Chinese Medicine for Cats and Dogs.* "It is a progressive form of immune imbalance." When a pet gets cancer, his immune system—including various vital organs—has usually been out of balance for a period of time.

One of Dr. Goldstein's mentors, Lawrence Burton, Ph.D., a renowned immune-system specialist, believes that 60 percent of cancers occur because of a genetically weak immune system.

"This genetic link is most obvious in dogs. For example, golden retrievers and rottweilers are at high risk for cancer because their popularity resulted in much inbreeding," says Dr. Goldstein. "I recently sent one of my patients, a golden retriever named Teddy, to the University of California, Davis, teaching hospital for a blood and medical evaluation. After the exam, Teddy's companion told me that of thirteen animals with cancer in the waiting room, twelve were golden retrievers. Goldens became the most popular breed in the early 1980s. In the wake of that popularity came indiscriminate breeding, resulting years later in multitudes of genetically weak, cancer-prone goldens."

Although it is still not known what causes most cancers, we do know what risk factors wreak havoc on the immune system. These immunity-zappers include too much sun; the presence of hormones in unneutered pets; feline leukemia virus (FeLV); feline immunodeficiency virus (FIV); and much more. Still, you can lower your pet's risk of getting cancer.

"The condition of the thymus gland and its associated lymphatic tissues and immunological functions is extremely important. If an animal can be kept in excellent health with good food, adequate exercise, access to fresh air and sunshine, and a stable emotional environment, this immune system will be strong," says Richard Pitcairn,

D.V.M., Ph.D., in his book *Dr. Pitcairn's Complete Guide to Natural Health for Dogs and Cats.* "Whereas a weaker animal might succumb to the effects of carcinogens, a strong one will more likely resist and detoxify them."

HISTORY OF CANCER IN PETS

Unfortunately, the surge in the number of deadly cancers merely conveys the magnitude of the pet-cancer epidemic. Indeed, the disease is becoming increasingly common in our time. Why is cancer skyrocketing? According to the American Animal Hospital Association, the reasons for increased cancer occurrences in animals are similar to the human paradox: as we live longer, our chance of developing some form of cancer increases. Before the 1970s, the average life span for a dog was seven to eight years, now it's ten to fifteen.

"Pets not only are becoming more susceptible to cancer because of increased age, they also share our environment and take in most of the same elements that contribute to cancer in humans," says Barbara Kitchell, head oncologist with the University of Illinois College of Veterinary Medicine in Champaign-Urbana, Illinois.

"Research suggests that environmental pollutants and chemicals in food are major factors in development and support of this group of diseases. The way I see it,

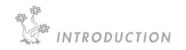
there are many factors that seem to cause cancer, but they don't take effect unless the individual is in a weakened, susceptible condition," says Dr. Pitcairn.

And to treat the cancer, holistic practitioners pay close attention to the immune system—and ultimately the pet's total body and spirit. That means this life-threatening disease is tackled in a *holistic* way.

HEALING YOUR PET WITH HOLISTIC MEDICINE

So what exactly is holistic medicine? "Holistic therapies tend not to seek single causes or cures, but to understand and treat disorder in the whole individual. Holistically minded practitioners do not divide diseases into separate components so much as they try to see how various disturbances in a person or animal are linked together," says Dr. Pitcairn.

"I have treated and consulted on thousands of cases of cancer and just about every variety. But unlike conventional practitioners, I pay the most attention to the immune system, not the cancer itself," adds Dr. Goldstein. "A strong immune system is able to resist cancer. So by charging up the immune system, which governs food metabolism, toxin elimination, and the destruction of foreign materials such as cancers, you can revitalize your animal's innate healing power."

And indeed, holistic vets use combinations of therapies to prevent cancer and sometimes even include conventional veterinary medicine to help treat and train the pet's body to heal itself.

Can cancer really be prevented? Yes, say holistic vets. Healthy lifestyle choices can help you guard your dog or cat against this life-threatening disease. So here is everything you wanted to know about how cancer can affect your pet from head to tail.

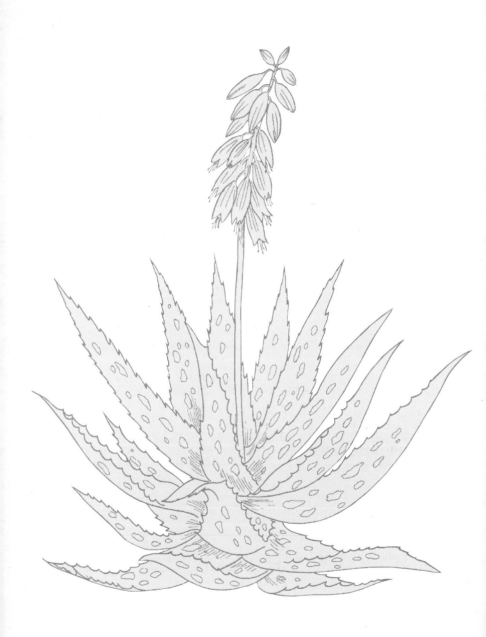

Cancer Awareness

HOW TO TELL IF YOUR PET HAS CANCER

Signs of cancer vary depending on the type of cancer. "Most lumps and bumps you feel on your dog's skin are harmless fatty tumors or fluid-filled cysts, but 80 percent of lumps or bumps on cats are malignant," says author Amy D. Shojai in her book *Competability*.

Dogs and cats can get the same types of cancers as each other but not always

DOGS AND CANCER

TYPE OF CANCER	OCCURRENCE	RANDOM FACTS
Skin cancer	The most common canine cancer	The least dangerous in dogs; common in older dogs; lumps are often benign
Breast (mammary) cancer	The second leading cause of cancer in dogs	Fifty percent of these tumors are malignant; spaying your pet before her first heat greatly reduces the risk
Lymphoma	The third most common canine cancer	Especially common in giant breeds
Bone cancer (osteosarcoma)	One of the most common canine cancers	Most commonly seen in large breed dogs; boxers, Saint Bernards, Great Danes, and wolfhounds have an increased risk; lameness may be an indication
Cancer of the mouth	Common in dogs	Many swellings are malignant; common in dogs with dark pigmentation inside their mouths
Hemangiosarcoma (cancer composed of blood vessels)	Common in golden retrievers	Usually starts in the spleen; first sign is sudden collapse

CATS AND CANCER

TYPE OF CANCER	OCCURRENCE	RANDOM FACTS
Lymphosarcoma (usually considered a part of feline leukemia complex)	The most common feline cancer	Nearly 90 percent of cases are caused by FeLV infection
Skin cancer	The second most common cancer in cats	Malignant in cats; can begin as a sun-induced lesion that may look like a slow-to-heal sore, usually on the bridge of the nose or tip of the ear
Cancer of the connective tissue (fibrosarcoma)	The third most common feline cancer	Often induced by vaccines. To counteract this, vets no longer vaccinate in just one spot.
Mammary cancer	Mammary tumors are common in cats	Mammary tumors are malignant 85 percent of the time; Siamese cats are twice as likely as other cat breeds to develop mammary cancer
Feline leukemia complex	Contagious among cats and occasionally causes true cancer	

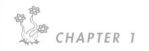

with the same frequency. According to the American Veterinary Medical Association (AVMA), some common types of cancers in dogs and cats are cancers of the skin, mammary tissue, lymphoid tissue, and bone.

SYMPTOMS TO LOOK FOR

Knowing that your pet is at high risk for developing cancer can be beneficial, and knowing the signs of cancer is even better. What may surprise you is that the symptoms of cancer in dogs and cats are usually the same as in people. And early detection is vital. A nine-year-old Labrador retriever named Max adopted John Cline, a certified public accountant, a few years ago. "Max would get soft lumps that came and went. One day, during the height of tax season, I was petting him and I felt a lump. It was hard," recalls John. "I had lost my mother to cancer, so despite my hectic work schedule I took him in." After a full chest X ray and biopsy, it was confirmed. Max had a malignant mast cell tumor. The outcome: The tumor was removed and Max is doing fine.

Successful treatment depends on the pet owner's ability to catch the symptoms early. "I usually tell people the best way to detect a tumor is just to pet their dog or cat a lot," says Ruthanne Chun, doctor of veterinary medicine and animal cancer specialist at Kansas State University. "If you happen to feel an abnormal bump or lump, or if the animal seems tender where it didn't used to be, then you ought to have it looked at." Because Max's owner detected the lump early and acted quickly, he was able to have the cancer removed and helped save Max's life.

First and foremost, the diagnosis of cancer must come from a veterinarian. Your doctor will gather evidence (X rays, ultrasound, blood tests, the physical appearance of the cancer, or the physical signs caused by the cancer) to verify that cancer is the verdict.

10 Warning Signs of Cancer in Pets

- Appetite loss
- Bad odor
- Bleeding or other discharge
- Difficulty breathing or eliminating
- Difficulty eating
- Exercise intolerance
- Ongoing lameness or stiffness
- Sores that don't heal
- Swelling that persists or continues to grow
- Weight loss

If your pet suffers from any of cancer's warning signs, consult with your veterinarian immediately.

The good news is: "...a diagnosis of cancer is not the death sentence it used to be. There are many methods of treatment, and there are new discoveries almost weekly," says Dr. Goldstein.

According to Dr. Pitcairn, treatments can have three outcomes: They can maintain a good quality of life during

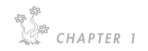

the time remaining; extend the life span beyond what is expected; or cure the condition by shrinking or obliterating the tumors.

Keep in mind, "Some cancers are more deadly and difficult to treat than others. An isolated skin cancer, for instance, is much less dangerous than a systemic lymph cancer. Treatment recommendations differ depending on the type and location of the cancer," adds Dr. Goldstein.

CHOOSING THE RIGHT NATURAL THERAPY

Treatment choices include the conventional—and some-times necessary—methods of chemotherapy, radiation therapy, cryosurgery (freezing), hyperthermia (artificially causing a fever), as well as alternative therapies such as immunotherapy.

Immunotherapy (drug therapy that stimulates the immune system) may help stave off cancer. "I have been using Immuno Augmentive Therapy (IAT) in combination with other holistic therapies to treat cancer since the mid-1970s. These therapies all work to balance the immune system, returning it to peak function," says Dr. Goldstein.

Like Dr. Goldstein, more and more holistic vets are fighting cancer by using IAT in combination with other conventional treatments and natural methods such as nutrition, vitamin-mineral supplements, homeopathy, herbs, and acupuncture.

Is one therapy any better than another? It's hard to say. "Conventional therapies all concentrate on killing the cancer directly. They miss the mark when it comes to the immune system. Surgery, chemotherapy, and radiation all suppress the immune system; however, they can be useful for what is termed 'debulking,'" says Dr. Goldstein. Debulking refers to reducing the mass of a tumor. In certain cases, debulking can buy more time for an immune enhancement program to take effect," adds Dr. Goldstein. And that's when the natural cancer therapies come into play. There are many ways to reinforce your pet's immune system. It's just a matter of what works best on the animal. In the next chapter, we'll examine the different therapies.

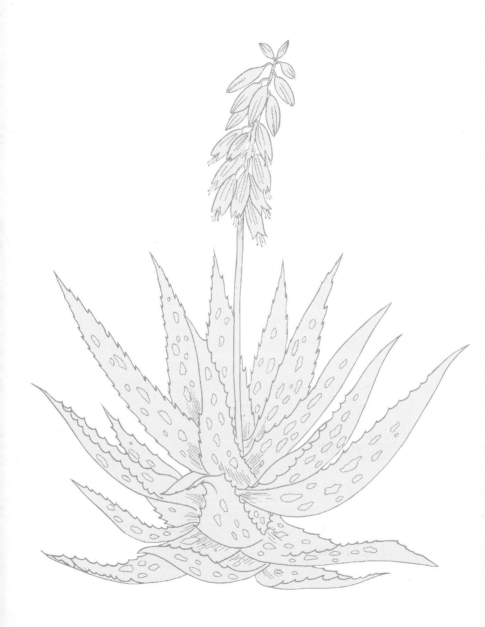

Natural therapies

By taking the plunge and trying the following therapies, you'll discover the holistic method that works best for your pet and learn how to control or cure cancer in the process! Be sure to consult with a vet who is knowledgeable in the field before beginning any type of treatment or dietary change.

THERAPY #1
THE HEALTH PROTECTION DIET

Del Goetz discovered a large lump on the chest of Pride,

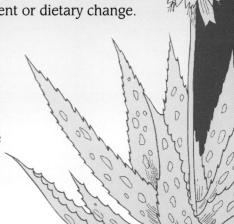

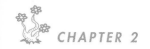

her nine-year-old Siberian husky. It scared her after all the dogs she's lost to cancer. After the biopsy, the vet notified Goetz that the husky had a malignant tumor. Without hesitation, she had the tumor surgically removed and changed the dog's diet. A researcher at heart, Del had suspected that the cancer that caused the deaths of her other three Siberian huskies was mainly due to ethoxyquin, a common preservative in soft-moist and other commercial pet food. She changed Pride's diet to an all-natural diet. After being carefully monitored for six years, the dog's lump has not returned. Today, Pride, at fifteen, eats a healthy, all-natural diet including home-prepared food.

Pat Kaufman's female basset hound, Freckles, is a cancer survivor too. She had to have one eye removed, however, and nearly died because of the disease. Kaufman put Freckles on an all-natural diet and fed her The Radiation Cocktail (a healthy drink that contains fresh juices) for a couple of weeks, and the dog's condition inproved.

You can't argue with success. "Diet is the number one cheapest and simplest way of preventing and fighting cancer," says Dr. Rivera. So go ahead. Make several changes to your pet's diet to guard against cancer, using our experts' health-protection, immunity-boosting nutrition plan.

Keep Pet Food Natural

Unnatural, processed commercial pet food can tax your pet's immune system. "This food contains ingredients, chemicals, toxins, and poisons that should not be consumed—and lacks ingredients that should be part of our pet's daily diet," wrote Dr. William Pollak in his article, "The Effects of a Natural vs. Commercial Pet Food Diet on the Wellness of Common Companion Animals—A Holistic Perspective," published in the *Journal of the American Holistic Veterinary Medical Association*, January 1997.

An all-natural diet can build up the immune system, which is an important step in preventing cancer or in moving toward a remission. A home-prepared diet containing fresh food is best. "When the entire diet is filled with fresh, whole food, the toxin level is much less from a physical perspective," says Dr. Pollak, who has a holistic practice in Fairfield, Iowa. "From a holistic perspective, the diet is providing what the body needs to naturally rid itself of cancer and enhance wellness." It's a back-to-nature route to optimal health.

Cook Your Pet's Meals

What's your best bet for ensuring your pet's health? Provide an all-natural, home-cooked diet that includes organic protein, whole grains, raw vegetables, and healthy oils. Because this type of diet is rich in vitamins, minerals,

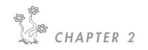

fiber, and living enzymes, it will support your pet's health.

To superenergize your pet, include "life force foods," says Dr. Goldstein. "Pets will not thrive on a diet made up of exclusively cooked foods. Raw vegetables may literally come to the rescue."

Many holistic vets recommend home-cooked dog food, but this may not always be practical for busy owners. Frozen raw food is the next best thing to home-cooked pet food. It's available at health food and pet stores, and it's supplemented with extra nutrients. Frozen raw food consists of mixed organ meats (heart, liver, lung, etc.) and muscle meat, raw vegetables, and occasionally grains. "Some of the diets [frozen food] may also contain additional glandular supplements, enzymes, garlic, and sea vegetables," notes Russell Swift, D.V.M., who specializes in homeopathy and nutrition in Tamarac, Florida.

Although no single food can prevent cancer, it's still important to feed your pet a variety of immunity-boosting, nutrient-dense foods to keep disease at bay.

Focus on Antioxidant-Rich Foods

Vegetables are chock-full of vitamins C and E and beta-carotene, which a dog's body converts into vitamin A and other carotenoids, all of which are antioxidants. (Cats can't convert beta-carotene to vitamin A, but the converted carotenoids are still good for them.) "These vitamins trap the free-radical molecules that cause normal cells to become cancerous," says Dr. Rivera. Antioxidants reduce the effects of free radicals and can calm inflammation and heal degenerative diseases such as cancer.

What's more, the phytochemicals known as indole-3-carbinols are suspected of having cancer-fighting abilities. "They, along with other phytochemicals—the chemicals in plant foods—support the body's immune functions," says Susan Wynn, D.V.M., of Marietta, Georgia, who specializes in scientifically based holistic medicine. To bolster your pet's immune system, Dr. Wynn suggests adding broccoli, cabbage, spinach, and carrots to your pet's home-cooked diet. It'll provide more nutrients and cancer-fighting fiber.

Boost Fiber Intake

For added cancer protection, holistic veterinarians combine an antioxidant-rich diet with high-fiber foods. According to Stanley Goldfarb, D.V.M., a holistic practitioner in San Rafael, California, a high-fiber diet helps prevent such woes as constipation, colitis, and inflammatory bowel disease—especially in cats after the first stage of lymphosarcoma of the intestine.

To lower your pet's risk of cancer, Dr. Rivera recommends increasing your pet's fiber intake to 16–17 percent a day. Your best food bets are vegetables, whole

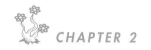
grains, and pumpkin. For the preparation and recommended quantity, please consult your veterinarian.

Low-Carbohydrate Diet

If you are living with a cancer-stricken pet, you might want to try another cancer-fighting diet strategy recommended by some holistic vets: a low-carbohydrate, home-prepared diet. This strategy is experimental, though. "The most important factor in feeding these animals is to reduce the carbohydrate level, because tumors 'steal' these nutrients from the patient, causing the tumors to grow faster while the patient loses weight," says Dr. Wynn. "The diet is formulated to reduce carbohydrate sources and provide very high-quality protein, and vegetables are added to provide fiber, vitamins, and minerals. A major source of energy is provided by fat in the diet." And fat may be the key cancer-fighting ingredient.

"Cancer cells cannot live off fat," points out Dr. Goldfarb. Both of these holistic vets recommend a diet for cancer patients that is low in carbs and moderate in protein to help reduce existing tumors. (See The Low-Carb Diet for Cancer Patients recipe pp.17–18).

Increase Powerful Nutrients

Dr. Goldstein has an immunity-boosting drink that is tailor-made for cancer patients. "This miraculous drink provides powerful—and I mean powerful—natural healing for just about any degenerative or chronic disease—including cancer," he says. Dr. Goldstein discovered this nutritional cocktail, called The Radiation Cocktail, when he was working with the cancer specialist Dr. Lawrence Burton. "Many of his human cancer patients had become weak from the radiation therapy. To rejuvenate their immune systems, they drank a special combination of concentrated nutrients, which we later adapted for animal use," says Dr. Goldstein.

According to Dr. Goldstein, this supercharged nutritional cocktail provides an abundance of digestible proteins. It triggers the body into manufacturing more immuno-proteins, which are necessary to fight disease. Other ingredients include cancer fighters such as beta-carotene; chlorophyll, which purifies the body; healing aloe vera; and vitamin E.

Cancer-Fighting Recipes

The following recipes are derived from "The Effects of a Natural vs. Commercial Pet Food Diet on the Wellness of Common Companion Animals—A Holistic Perspective" by William Pollak, D.V.M. Consult your vet before feeding the following diets to ensure your pet is getting the correct amount.

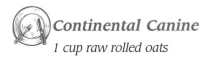

Continental Canine
1 cup raw rolled oats

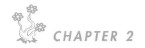

> *3 eggs (shells crushed and baked at 350° F for 12 minutes)*
> *1 tsp bonemeal or calcium/magnesium powder*
> *½ cup cottage cheese*
> *1 cup raw vegetable (whatever is on hand)*
> *1 cup raw chopped meat (chicken, turkey, or beef)*

Bring 2 cups of water to a boil. Add raw oats, cover, and cook 2 minutes. Turn off heat and let stand about 10 minutes. Stir in remaining ingredients. Mix in some brewer's or nutritional yeast, lecithin, and olive oil.

Feed 1½ cups per 35 lbs of dog per day. Needs vary based on activity level and age of dog.

Chewy Cat Cuisine

> *1 cup cornmeal or oatmeal*
>
> *2 eggs*
>
> *2 lbs (4 cups) raw or lightly cooked ground turkey or chicken (or lean chuck, heart, hamburger, liver giblets, fish, or other lean meats)*
>
> *4 Tbs vitamin/mineral powder*
>
> *2 Tbs bonemeal or chopped, softened, or ground eggshells*
>
> *2 Tbs olive oil or butter (or 1 Tbs each)*
>
> *15,000 IU vitamin A*
>
> *200 IU vitamin E*
>
> *600 mg taurine (optional)*
>
> *1 tsp fresh vegetable, ground, include fresh with each meal*

Bring 4 cups (1 quart) of water to a boil. Add the cornmeal or oatmeal. When thoroughly blended, cover and simmer on low 10–15 minutes. Stir in eggs and oil or butter. Mix in remaining ingredients. Serve fresh for two days. Feed ¼ to ½ cup per day for a medium-size cat. Divide the rest into meal-size portions and freeze.

The Low-Carb Diet for Cancer Patients

This diet is experimental. The proportions are not balanced for long-term use, so stay in touch with your veterinarian throughout the course of treatment for instructions or modifications.

	Dogs	**Cats**
Meat	*30-50%*	*40-60%*
Vegetables	*30-40%*	*20-30%*
Grains	*0-10%*	*0-10%*
Bonemeal	*½ tsp per cup of food*	*½ tsp per cup of food*
Extra-strength Marine-lipid Capsules (omega-3 fatty acids)	*1 extra-strength capsule per day*	*1 regular-strength capsule per day*

Protein sources should include eggs, chicken, turkey, fish, and occasionally lamb. Raw meat is preferable, but if the animal is receiving chemotherapy, the immune suppression makes bacterial contamination a danger.

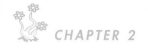

Cook the meat rare, or decontaminate the outside by placing the meat in boiling water for 5 minutes.

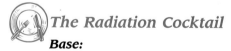 A variety of vegetables should be provided. "Leafy, green vegetables, carrots, and anything from the broccoli family have an anticancer effect in humans and probably in animals, too," says Dr. Nancy Scanlan, a holistic practitioner in California.

Grains should be complex carbohydrates such as wheat, oats, barley, rice, and corn. Add them in the form of cooked oatmeal, pasta, and brown rice.

Animals eating home-prepared diets should always receive a multivitamin-mineral supplement as well as bonemeal to balance phosphorus and calcium ratio.

The following dietary supplement was invented by Dr. Bob Goldstein.

The Radiation Cocktail

Base:

¼ cup of distilled or filtered pure water

½ cup raw organic calf liver (fresh and blended) or 2 organic raw egg yolks (no whites)

1 tsp powdered dulse or kelp

1 Tbs nutritional yeast (unprocessed containing B vitamins)

1 tsp organic apple cider vinegar

½ tsp ground rosemary

400 IU vitamin E

Fresh juices (add just before feeding):

½ cup of organic carrot juice (freshly extracted)

1 Tbs parsley juice (freshly extracted)

1 tsp aloe vera juice

In a blender, gently mix all the ingredients on the lowest-speed possible. Use fresh juices because they contain live enzymes. Make a couple of days' supply of the base and add the fresh juices just before feeding. Force-feed animals who aren't eating. Don't overfeed and cause vomiting. For cats and small- to medium-size dogs, feed 2 to 5 Tbs per day. Large and giant breeds (50 lbs and larger) can take up to 10 Tbs. Ingredients are available at health food stores.

THERAPY #2
DIETARY SUPPLEMENTS

Healthy dogs and cats need extra nutrition "because of the pollution and stress common to modern life," while less healthy dogs and cats need vitamins and minerals to speed along the recovery process, explains Dr. Pitcairn.

Adding nutrition-packed food supplements, such as bonemeal and vegetable oil, can help pets who aren't in

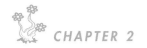
the best of health, notes Dr. Pitcairn. Plus, supplements fortify the diet with vitamins and minerals that are often lost from fresh foods during storage and cooking.

In addition, more Western vets are touting vitamins, minerals, and antioxidants to fight cancer. "It is much easier to use vitamins and nutritional supplements, along with a good diet, as a *preventive measure* before the immune system comes under attack," says Dr. Schwartz. "Once the immune system is out of balance, supplementation becomes an essential adjunct to life."

To maintain good health, holistic vets recommend good quality natural vitamins. "Synthetic, bargain supplements aren't assimilated and metabolized well, and can even cause adverse reactions in your animal," says Dr. Goldstein. You can get all-natural, immunity-boosting nutritional supplements at a health food store.

Cancer-Preventing Nutrients

A diet rich in antioxidant foods and nutritional supplements may help prevent cancer. Here's a look at popular cancer-fighting vitamins and supplements and the protection they offer. For the right dosage or quantity, please consult your veterinarian. The following supplements help prevent the spread of cancer.

 Ester C: "Cancer is an immune-deficiency disease,

CANCER FIGHTERS

ANTIOXIDANT	WHAT IT DOES	BEST FOOD BETS
Beta-carotene (precursor of vitamin A)	Converts to vitamin A in dog's liver; reduces effects of free radicals	Carrots
Other carotenoids	Results are often better using a combination of carotenoids, rather than beta-carotene alone	Green, leafy vegetables
Vitamin A	Destroys carcinogens; high doses can be toxic	Cod liver oil
Vitamin C	Boosts protective white blood cells; helps heal skin and intestinal lining	Broccoli, brussels sprouts
Vitamin E	Helps prevent free-radical damage to cells, which can lead to abnormal cell growth	Olive oil, egg yolk, wheat germ
Selenium	Fights cancer by repairing cells and preventing cell mutation, which boosts the immune system	Chicken

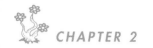

and vitamin C strengthens the immune system. When the diagnosis of a serious, life-threatening cancer is made, add vitamin C to the program at a dose just below bowel tolerance. Purchase vitamin C as ascorbic acid tablets or in a powder form called sodium ascorbate," says Dr. Goldstein. Sodium ascorbate, or ester C, is buffered vitamin C. If your pet gets runny stool, decrease the dosage.

Fish oils: Dr. Goldfarb says that these oils are high in omega-3 fatty acids, which help fight the spread of cancer cells. Your best choices are salmon, mackerel, and sardines, which are good sources of fish oils because they have the highest fat content and provide more omega-3 factors than other fishes.

Essential fatty acids: "The oils that are found in olive and vegetable oil convert into prostaglandins . . . which stimulate the immune system and help battle cancer," says Dr. Schwartz. They also rid the body of toxins and regulate autoimmune diseases. "Too much vegetable oil can be pro-oxidant, so limit its use," says Dr. Scanlan. "Olive and fish oils don't have this effect."

Cartilage: Cartilage (which has no blood vessels) is thought to wall off and decrease the blood supply to cancerous cells, thereby inhibiting their growth. Although cartilage can be somewhat expensive, new discoveries show that it helps reduce cancerous tumors when taken orally. "I recommend cartilage for cancer patients—both shark and bovine cartilage," says Dr. Goldstein.

THERAPY #3
ANTICANCER HERBS
AND HOMEOPATHY

In addition to a power-packed diet for your cancer-afflicted pet, research shows that when herbs and homeopathic remedies team up, they create a superpowerful weapon in the war against cancer.

For starters, herbs can help nourish a dog or cat after chemotherapy or radiation treatment, which leave a pet weak or thin. Herbs also are used to treat pain. Dr. Schwartz explains the Chinese belief that pain stems from blockage of *qi* (pronounced "chee"), or circulation, along the pathways of energy called meridians. "When herbs are prescribed, they address the blockage problem, and also help to strengthen the bones and the tissues surrounding the painful area." Here are six cancer-fighting herbs (work with your vet to find the proper dosage for your pet):

Astragalus: This root (available in an extract that is given orally) is rich in flavonones, which help circulation

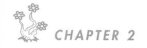

and blood production. This Chinese herb is becoming well known in the West for helping to treat cancer. "Because it enhances circulation," says Dr. Schwartz, "it helps prevent stagnation that can cause tumors to form. Astragalus also contains polysaccharides, which help to inhibit tumor formation." Astragalus has been proven to boost strength, stamina, and digestion after chemotherapy and radiation treatment—and even increases survival rates in cancer patients after these treatments.

Goldenseal: According to Dr. Pitcairn, this herb is good for treating any type of cancer, especially if the cancer is associated with weight loss. Goldenseal can damage the liver so extra vitamin B complex is advised during prolonged use. Dr. Scanlan recommends giving Goldenseal orally two to three times a day for three weeks, stopping for one week, then continuing again for three weeks.

Essiac: Essiac's cancer-fighting punch comes from herbs such as sheep sorrel, burdock root, slippery elm bark, and rhubarb root, which together make this a strong herbal tonic and detoxifier. It's an energy-boosting oral treatment that works well with other remedies. Essiac can be found at health food stores, labeled as "essiac" or mixed with a few other herbs in "Flor-Essence."

Aloe vera juice: According to Dr. Goldstein, aloe vera juice can be used internally or externally to purify the body and aid in detoxification. Mix 1 tablespoon into 2 cups of water and add it to your pet's drinking water or rub the undiluted gel right on the tumor if it's visible.

Ganoderma and maitake mushrooms: New research in Asia has shown that eating these dried herbal mushrooms may help halt or delay tumor growth and stop the spread of certain tumors.

Garlic: This herb helps protect cells from cancer-causing agents. People and pets get both preventive and therapeutic benefits from eating fresh or extracted garlic. Research shows that it slows the progression of an existing tumor cell and blocks the formation of new tumor cells. Use cautiously with cats; too much can cause a type of anemia.

Homeopathic Remedies

Sarge, a nine-year-old springer spaniel, suffered bleeding from the nose. She was taken to a conventional vet for tests. The diagnosis was that cancer had developed inside the nose of the dog. Although her type of disease is inoperable, it has not spread because the cancer-stricken dog was put on a new nutritional program and began sil-

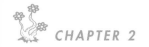

icea homeopathic treatment. Several weeks later, Sarge was free of symptoms.

Homeopathy, such as the silicea remedy given to Sarge, works on the premise of "like cures like," and homeopathic medicines contain very small amounts of substances that would cause similar symptoms to the ones a patient is enduring if given to a well animal. You find success when a homeopathic remedy fits an individual pet's cancer symptoms.

"We use homeopathy as another alternative therapy to try and help shrink tumors and help stimulate the immune system," says holistic and conventional vet Shawn Messonnier of Plano, Texas. Bear in mind that the choice of treatment and dosage must be made by a doctor of homeopathy.

Homeopathic remedies are usually available in sugar tablets. If your pet won't eat tablets, you can dissolve them in 1 tsp distilled water. Shake up the solution and use an eyedropper to give orally. According to Dr. Pitcairn, the following homeopathic remedies can be used as treatments for cancer patients. He advises to start with using herbal goldenseal and homeopathic *Thuja occidentalis* first.

Thuja occidentalis 30C: This treatment is preferably used at the outset of cancer because it gets rid of the influence of prior vaccinations that may stimulate the growth of tumors. Give one tablet every other day, indefinitely or until the cancer is gone.

Natrum muriaticum 6C (NaCl): This homeopathic tissue salt is most helpful to cats who have solid tumors or lymphosarcoma, especially those cats suffering with appetite problems.

Silicea 6C: Silicea 6C is most helpful to dogs who have solid tumors or lymphosarcoma but is especially effective in dogs who have ravenous appetites but are losing weight.

Conium maculatum 6C: This poison hemlock is used for animals who have very hard tumors.

Phosphorus 6C: This homeopathic remedy is used for tumors that tend to bleed persistently.

THERAPY #4
ACUPUNCTURE

Another popular natural weapon for cancer protection is the ancient Chinese art of acupuncture. It involves the insertion of fine needles into specific areas of the body,

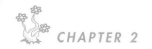
which stimulates nerve fibers and releases pain-relieving endorphins, those feel-good hormones.

Amazing research has shown that certain acupoints (points on the body where the needles are inserted) rev up white and red blood cells and boost the immune response, which rids toxins from the body. How? "Acupuncture does this by causing the body to set up a chain of events that releases such substances as hormones, neurotransmitters, ion exchanges, antibodies, antihistamines, and interferon. These cell transmitters ease the movement of the abnormal cells across the cell walls into the blood and lymph system to be removed from the body," explains Dr. Schwartz.

Michelle Tilghman, D.V.M., a holistic vet in Stone Mountain, Georgia, who sees cancer patients daily, uses acupuncture mainly for pain relief. It's especially therapeutic for dogs and cats who are showing musculoskeletal pain, which is a side effect to the cancer. This, in turn, helps improve the quality of a cancer patient's life.

Consider one golden retriever, for example. He had an inoperable tumor in his bladder. Rather than allow the canine to suffer or resort to euthanasia, his owners opted for acupuncture treatment to relieve pain. The treatment also bought time. The dog lived much longer than expected.

What You Can Do at Home

Pam, a dog owner, knows that fighting cancer can be a winning battle. One day she found a lump on the chest of her Akita-mix, Makeetah. "He has fatty tumors that I was told to monitor that had changed shape and hardened. A biopsy indicated that Makeetah had a grade-one mast cell tumor," she recalls.

After surgery, Pam followed an immune-boosting at-home plan to keep Makeetah healthy and hopefully cancer-free. While Pam provided a healthy dog chow of premium lamb, rice,

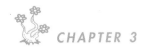
and vegetarian food, plus fresh foods and supplements, she was advised by Dr. Goldstein to go a step further.

She needed to be on the alert for any stress that would make Makeetah emotionally upset and avoid vaccinations because of their potential to suppress the immune system. Also, she needed to get Makeetah physically examined annually and ask her vet for a routine blood exam that included a complete blood count, complete chemistries, and a thyroid test. It was important to meet with a holistic vet to set up a program that addressed any nutrient deficiencies and to have the dog's blood looked at from an immune-system perspective.

Like Makeetah, more and more dogs and cats are becoming cancer survivors because their pet owners are doing their holistic homework. Here, Drs. Pitcairn, Schwartz, and Goldstein provide ten at-home preventive strategies to help guard your pet against cancer:

TEN NONDIET WAYS
TO PREVENT CANCER

1. Provide only pure water. Tap water is often polluted with toxic chemicals such as lead, arsenic, and nitrates. Holistic vets strongly advise using a good-quality water purifier. "...By getting fresh water (bottled or distilled), you can rejuvenate your pet because it flushes toxins from the body and contributes to the feeling of well-being," says Dr. Goldstein.

If you decide to buy a water purifier, keep in mind that "although initially costlier than bottled water, it is much cheaper in the long run, costing only pennies a gallon," says Dr. Pitcairn.

2. If your pet already has cancer, avoid all vaccinations. Vaccinations can stress your pet's immune system. Recently, one cat owner found this out. Her nine-year-old cat, Sam, contracted a disease called vaccine-induced fibrosarcoma. This is a fatal cancer for cats that develops at the site of repeated vaccine injections, say holistic vets.

Sam was one of the lucky ones. Two thousand dollars later, the tumor on his shoulder was gone. Today, Sam is in remission and looks 100 percent better.

"For cancer patients, at the very least, avoid vaccinations during treatment because they will counteract any positive and immune-enhancing effects of your home-support program," says Dr. Goldstein. Ask your vet about the homeopathic remedy *Thuja occidentalis* 30C, which removes the immune-suppressing effects of vaccinations.

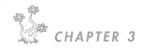

3. Avoid indoor pollution. Keep your pet away from cigarette smoke. Studies show that secondhand smoke contains hundreds of toxic chemicals that can cause lung cancer in humans. It hasn't been shown to be as much of a problem for animals, yet vets still recommend that you avoid exposing your pet to it.

Ventilate your house well to reduce indoor air pollution. Grow houseplants that filter the air such as philodendrons, spider plants, aloe vera, chrysanthemums, and gerbera daisies, and keep the plants out of your pet's reach. Don't use chemicals such as pesticides and household cleaners around the house. Seek out natural products.

4. Avoid contaminated water. Keep your pet away from street puddles, which can contain cancer-causing toxins such as hydrocarbons and asbestos dust from brakes.

You should change your pet's water daily. Keep the bowl clean and in a place protected from dust and debris. "Most of all," says Dr. Pitcairn, "make it available so that your pet will not be tempted to drink from a contaminated puddle, creek, or pond."

5. Keep your pet away from electromagnetic radiation. Be careful that your pet is not exposed to many environmental sources of electromagnetic radiation such as power lines close to the house and areas with a lot of electrical outlets.

Remember to keep your pet from resting on or near a color TV set, as many holistic vets believe that all radiation effects are cumulative in the body. Keep Fido and Fluffy away from radios, microwaves, and computer terminals, too.

6. Don't use unnatural flea products on your pet. Did you know that flea collars, sprays, and shampoos are full of poisons? Instead of chemical insecticides, use natural and less-toxic methods of flea control such as natural flea shampoos, vacuuming frequently, and combing your pet with a flea comb. Pyrethins are a natural means of flea control. D-limonen and other citrus-based methods can be used on dogs (there is evidence of toxicity in cats). Putting borates, salt, or diatomaceous earth into carpet is effective for indoor flea control.

7. Do not allow your pet to ride in the back of a pickup truck. Along with the danger of being thrown out of the truck, your pet will be susceptible to inhaling toxic car fumes and smog. Let your dog or cat get fresh air either by way of a park, beach, or your backyard. For indoor cats, open up a screened window and let your feline get a breath of fresh outdoor air.

8. Keep your pet away from pesticides and herbicides on lawns and plants. A report by The National Cancer Institute found that dogs whose owners used a common weed killer had twice the rate of lymphoma as dogs whose owners did not use it.

Stay clear of house and garden pesticides, and get rid of pesky insects naturally; or seek out the least-toxic products. There are also nontoxic, organic products available.

9. Keep your pet stress-free. Stress is emotional imbalance caused by anger, frustration, or anxiety. These emotions overwork the liver, where they can stagnate and create tumors, according to Dr. Schwartz.

High anxiety in pets happens for a variety of reasons: neglect, a multiple animal household, an owner going away on vacation, or an owner going through a divorce. Whatever triggers stress in your dog or cat, tune in and help your pet chill out.

Try some de-stressing methods such as: maintaining a regular pet routine (including feeding times and playtimes); massaging your pet; being in tune to your pet's needs; looking for stress signals (from appetite changes to excessive barking); keeping peace in a multipet household; and providing tender loving care.

10. Exercise your dog or cat on a regular basis. Research shows that canine and feline fitness not only strengthens immunity to chronic disease such as cancer but is also essential for optimal health and well-being.

"Sustained, vigorous use of the muscles stimulates all tissues and increases blood circulation. Blood vessels dilate and blood pressure rises. As a result, tissues become oxygenated, which helps to clean the cells of toxins. Digestive glands secrete their fluids better, and the bowels move more easily," says Dr. Pitcairn.

Some activities that you can enjoy with your pooch to get fit together are bicycling, hiking, jogging, in-line skating, and walking (at least twenty minutes a day). Some fun feline workouts are hiding games (with a bed sheet, tented paper, or paper bag), playing with interactive cat toys or windup toys, scratching a pad or post, and walking your cat on a harness and leash.

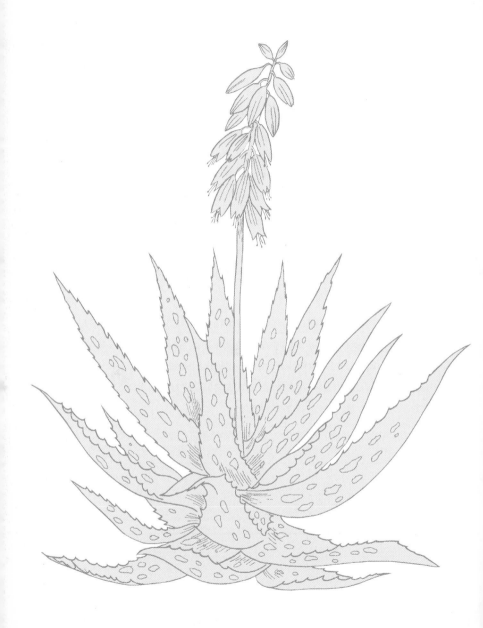

What's to Come in the future

Two years ago, Amber, a ten-year-old golden retriever–mix, stopped barking. Her owners, Adrienne and Frank Crognale, took her to the vet, and she was diagnosed with a deadly cancer in the left tonsil and the larynx. A biopsy confirmed the diagnosis of squamous cell carcinoma, an extremely aggressive cancer that often quickly invades other parts of the body. The pet owners' vet recommended chemotherapy, drugs, and radiation.

Amber's companions took another route instead. First, the tumor in Amber's throat was

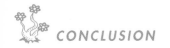

removed surgically. Then, after doing a blood test that examined the immune system, the prescription was a series of homeopathic and glandular remedies, vitamins, minerals, and enzymes—an entire program focused on boosting her sluggish glands. Six months later, Amber was healed and looking great.

This move toward holistic care in the prevention and treatment of cancer will be linked to a new way of thinking when pet owners realize it's smarter to keep a pet healthy than to wait until she gets ill. Once "converted to the holistic approach to pet care, it is difficult to look at it any other way. A new preventive emphasis, which means going back to the basics, will be the wave of the future," says S. Allen Price, D.V.M, a holistic veterinarian and nutrition specialist in Birmingham, Alabama.

"Most of today's practitioners use alternative medicines allopathically—to confront disease," says Randy Kidd, D.V.M., in Kansas City, Kansas. "Practitioners will ultimately have to learn to use the alternative medicines in their natural manner—relying on the patient's innate body, mind, and spirit itself to return to a state of health."

In the upcoming years, there will be an increase in holistic health care, and pet owners such as Amber's companions will become more involved on a one-to-one basis with their pet's well-being. It will be common to do whatever it takes, from home-cooking to homeopathy, to keep our dogs and cats healthy, happy, and cancer-free.

THE IN-HOME COMPUTER REVOLUTION

By 2020, veterinarians will view surgery as a last resort for treating cancer and other deadly diseases. Instead, a new and improved game plan to ward off illness will keep chronic diseases, such as cancer, and their effects at a minimum. "Ultimately, people and pets will be able to heal themselves and to become and stay healthy without much intervention, especially on the physical level," says Christina Chambreau, D.V.M., a homeopathic veterinarian in Baltimore, Maryland.

Also by 2020, people will be able to stay healthier via telemedicine with a virtual doctor who appears on a computer or TV wall screen, according to Michio Kaku, a New York–based theoretical physicist and author of *Visions*. This "virtual doctor" may regularly diagnose and prescribe preventive treatment to ward off illness. Pets may easily be included in this computerized technology. Perhaps a tiny computer nestled in your pet's collar will keep track of your pet, warn her not to jump on the TV, and monitor her well-being.

Another scientific breakthrough by the year 2020, according to Dr. Kaku, will be the development of the Internet into a resource that can tune into the wisdom of

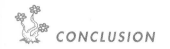

experts around the planet to educate us. Certainly, such a system would teach pet owners more about their animals' care and behavior, thus improving their health and happiness. What's more, computers may act as an alert system to help prevent health problems such as cancer before it's too late.

ALTERNATIVE THERAPIES ON THE RISE

The increase in cancer rates in both humans and pets has contributed to the advancement of traditional treatments and natural treatments. According to holistic experts, new cancer-fighters not mentioned in this book will be available or more widely used in the future. These include ozone therapy; inositol hexaphosphate (IP6)—a substance derived from fiber; and soy-based pet foods.

For humans, integrated-medicine clinics for chronic diseases are hot; and for pets, prototypes are in the cards. "It is already becoming more common to administer acupuncture during surgical pet procedures," says Gregory L. Tilford, herbalist and CEO of Animals' Apawthecary. Holistic experts predict that veterinary practices of the future will include both traditional and alternative therapies for cancer treatment under the same roof.

Just ask Jordan Kocen, D.V.M., M.S., a certified veterinary acupuncturist who joined the staff at South Paws

Veterinary Referral Center in Springfield, Virginia, two years ago. Although his practice is limited to holistic medicine—acupuncture, homeopathy, and Chinese herbal medicine—the other specialty practices at the facility include surgery, internal medicine, and oncology. Dr. Kocen predicts that veterinary medicine will follow this model of incorporating nonconventional therapies into the general practice of medicine. "Many conditions tend to respond best to a particular form of alternative therapy and many respond best to a combination of holistic with conventional."

A NEW WAVE OF SELF-RELIANCE

Both veterinarians and pet owners are changing the way they view health care—and it's for the better. "The biggest shift, which I see happening already, is that people are taking personal responsibility for their animal's health," says Dr. Chambreau. "People are less willing to accept what experts are telling them and are researching for themselves what makes their animals feel better."

Like Adrienne and Frank Crognale, countless other pet owners are learning that they can take responsibility to research holistic remedies and help their pets heal naturally. With the aid of holistic medicine, we are often able to keep ourselves and our pets living healthier and longer lives.

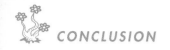
LIFE GOES ON

Bear in mind, a diagnosis of cancer is not always a sign that your pet's days are numbered. Many types of cancer are curable, and the length of your pet's life can be increased and its quality improved with an immune-boosting, fresh, natural diet, plus herbs, exercise, and other holistic therapies.

To this the author can personally attest. Gandolf, her fearless seventeen-year-old cat, fell victim to a feline sub-cutaneous mast cell malignant tumor that can exhibit unexpected aggressive behavior. She was advised to have the tumor removed as soon as possible. After the operation, she kept her "Rock of Gibraltar" on a diet free of artificial colors and flavors, put a stop to all vaccinations, and kept him indoors in a mellow, chemical-free household.

As a result, Gandolf enjoyed Orey and his feline companion, Alex, for another year and a half.

Above all, each animal handled with a holistic approach—Pride, Max, Makeetah, Amber, and others—experienced that cancer is far from being terminal. Your pet, too, can arrive at that point.

For a listing of holistic veterinarians in your area, contact:
American Holistic Veterinary Medical Association
2214 Old Emmorton Road, Bel Air, MD 21015
(410) 569-0795

Much of the research and information on natural medicine comes from a variety of sources that can be difficult to find. While the amount of written research is growing, a lot of the information still can be found only in unpublished sources. In addition to using the conventional sources such as books, magazines, and veterinary journals, the author interviewed holistic and conventional veterinarians and researched several unpublished sources including news releases and articles from the Internet. Following are sources in which you can find more information on cancer.

Books and Magazines

Kaku, Michio. *Visions*. New York: Doubleday, 1997.

Orey, Cal. "Pet Predictions for the Year 2020," *Natural Pet*. March/April 1998.

Orey, Cal. "Anticancer Diet," *Natural Pet*. July/August 1997.

Pitcairn, Richard, H., D.V.M., and Susan Hubble Pitcairn. *Dr. Pitcairn's Complete Guide to Natural Health for Dogs and Cats*. Emmaus, PA: Rodale Press, 1995.

Pollak, William, D.V.M., "The Effects of a Natural vs. Commercial Pet Food Diet on the Wellness of Common Companion Animals," *Journal of the American Holistic Veterinary Medical Association*. January 1997.

Schwartz, Cheryl, D.V.M., *Four Paws: A Guide to Chinese Medicine for Cats and Dogs*. Berkeley, CA: Celestial Arts, 1996.

Shojai, Amy, D. *Competability: A Practical Guide to Building a Peaceable Kingdom Between Cats and Dogs.* Three Rivers Press, 1998.

Singin' The Kerry Blues. The Kerry Blue Terrier Club of Northern California, November 1997.

Internet and Other Sources

"Animal Cancer," (http://www.avma.org/care4pets/ancancr.html) American Veterinary Medical Association, 1998.

Goldstein, Bob, V.M.D., and Susan Goldstein. *The Goldstein Program for Healthy Animals: Twenty-One Days to Better Health.* Pamphlet

Goldstein, Bob, V.M.D., and Susan Goldstein. *Love of Animals* newsletter. To subscribe to the newsletter or to receive volumes, pamphlets, and other pet-related information from Dr. Bob Goldstein and Susan Goldstein, call Earth Animal at 1-800-211-6365.

"Humans Are Not the Only Victims: Owners Should Be Aware that Pets Are Susceptible to Cancer," (http://www.newss.ksu.edu/WEB/News/NewsReleases/listpetcancer.html) Kansas State University News Services, Thursday, August 7, 1997.

"Increase in Pet Cancer Rate Bridges Gap to Human Treatment." American Animal Hospital Association. News Release, 1995.

ABOUT THE AUTHOR

Cal Orey, a freelance writer based in northern California, has a master's degree in English from San Francisco State University. In the past decade, she has written hundreds of articles about human and pet health in many national magazines, including *Dog Fancy* and *Natural Dog*. She owns a nine-year-old Brittany spaniel, Dylan, and a look-alike thirteen-year-old laid-back cat named Alex. Cal dedicates this book to her cat Gandolf, a companion she had for nearly twenty years, and to her father, who died of cancer. Her father's and beloved pet's spirits remain a source of her creativity and inspiration.

ABOUT THE VETERINARIAN

Dr. Nancy Scanlan graduated from University of California, Davis, in 1970. She has used nutritional therapy since her senior year there. She has been certified in veterinary acupuncture since 1988 and has taught animal health and animal science for ten years. Dr. Scanlan regularly writes articles for various pet-related magazines. She currently practices holistic-only medicine in California, using acupuncture, nutritional therapy, Chinese and Western herbs, trigger point therapy, and Chiropractic. If you are interested in getting in touch with Dr. Scanlan, contact the American Holistic Veterinary Medical Association.

For more about natural pet care, look for *Natural Cat* and *Natural Dog* magazines at pet stores and selected newsstands.

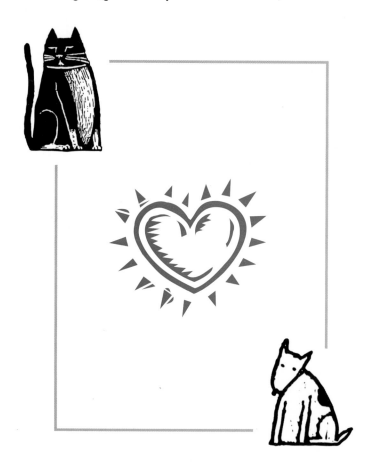